# PREVENTATIVE MAINTENANCE
## FOR LIVING A LIFE OF HEALTH AND WELLNESS

RJ SMITH

Copyright © 2019 . RJ Smith

Parchment Global Publishing
4152 Barnett St., Philadelphia, PA 19135
www.parchmentglobalpublishing.com

ISBN: 978-1-950981-38-0 (sc)
ISBN: 978-1-950981-39-7 (e)

All rights reserved. No part of this book may be reproduced, stored, or transmitted by any means—whether auditory, graphic, mechanical, or electronic—without written permission of both publisher and author, except in the case of brief excerpts used in critical articles and reviews. Unauthorized reproduction of any part of this work is illegal and is punishable by law.

This program is for you if you have...

- ➢ Excess weight - if you have lost it or need to lose it;
- ➢ Poor health - to make the changes that will put you on the right path;
- ➢ Good health - this program will maintain it, as you will be able also.

Prevent the return of the weight so you can and will maintain what you have accomplished.

I am a man of 88 who maintains my good health. I know the answer to the question "What is my health worth?"

Priceless!

And you will find the same answer, as this will work for you at any age, and this will put you on a path to be

The best you can be!

Here are some very good ideas and tools for reaching your goals and maintaining them - for your entire family - even in your own home.

Brain - Body Connection

The best-kept health care secret anywhere, healing messages to all parts of your body.

No drugs, no surgery. More than 100 different health problems have responded to this procedure. I have seen this up close, as I have had this procedure. Find out what to look for. It could do wonders for you. Yes, you can maintain your newfound health and look forward to A life of health and wellness.

See how I, a man of 88, uses enjoyable exercises and nutritional meals to make a healthy individual. The exercises, some of which are used by astronauts, are things that your whole family will enjoy, even in your own house. You will be able to reach your goals and, most importantly, maintain them as I have.

We realize that to be healthy people we need to be active people, as that is part of our makeup. Sure, we can become slender, as there are many products that will help us achieve that goal. However, if we continue to be inactive, we will only be slender, unhealthy people, and soon, the weight will return. Getting your body in shape and then maintaining it, that is what this book is about. It will give you a healthy life with some longevity to it. To find the keys you need for your health and wellness, I have some good ideas for you to read about and put into practice. Yes, you can be on your way to be the best you that can be. This can be life changing, for sure, and lead to a life of health and wellness.

Remember, it's never too late to start taking care of yourself. It is a wonderful feeling to be as healthy as you can be. So get up and get moving. You will find that, when you are healthy and feeling good, all aspect of your life will be so much better, and you will be able to handle everyday stress in a calm manner. Once you gain confidence, you can see that we, ourselves, can truly be our own best prescription.

See how this works for you.

HELLO

I am a man of 88 years who has so far lived a full life. I had been married for forty-eight wonderful years when my wife suddenly passed away, which was a huge loss for me and my family. I have two great daughters and two wonderful grandchildren who I'm fortunate to see most every month.

I'm so very blessed as I have a wonderful lady friend, and we have a great time together.

I really have a deep concern for how overweight and out of shape we are throughout this great country of ours, since I have 88 years from which to draw some knowledge, I want to let people know what I do to maintain my good health and wellness.

Hopefully, you will find some value and encouragement in this story. I have seen up close and in person what exercise and eating the proper foods can do for your blood pressure, cholesterol, and overall wellbeing. By changing some things, I am now a very healthy person, and I continue to do the necessary things to maintain a healthy lifestyle.

The ability to maintain is what we are searching for; it is the key to our continued well-being.

"Find out how this man of 88 yrs. makes this work and how he maintains his good health"

"A deep concern about how overweight and out of shape" "Find encouragement"

"You are in control to maintain what you accomplish"

By RJSMITH

I think most of us realize that we need to change the poor habits we have developed. Look in the mirror and encourage yourself, love ones, and friends to look after themselves by eating and exercising properly. We need to keep in mind that we have to get up and get moving, and then we will be on our way to the best we can be.

"Talk about it with family and friends " "no, not what we are about" "Just a scratch pad works fine" "it's easy-you can do it"

I want to be perfectly clear. This is not about some magic pill that will drop pounds off of you without doing or changing anything or that will allow you to be a couch potato.

No, that's not what this book is about at all.

This is really about maintaining a healthy lifestyle after reaching your goals by doing the same things on a regular basis. Think about it. Many of us have tried a diet at some time in our life, and we either lose sight of our goals or tell ourselves that we are doing OK. Pretty soon, it is over. So, yes, we have to write down in our log what we have to eat at each meal and what we did and how much time we spent each day doing it. Looking at what you accomplished last week really will tell you to either get with it or that you did a good job for yourself. Seeing the figures tells you everything. Yes, you most likely will have to change your eating habits, including cutting down the portions and exercising daily. You need to make it a habit to make this work for you. But you can do it. Just think—a healthy lifestyle. Time is of the essence as people have busy lives. But if you want to be around for your children and grandchildren, you had better look in the mirror and talk with that person about where you are heading.

Find out from your primary care physician just what kind of shape you are in and what your plan should be to change the problems you have. You can be struck down at any time, even at a young age, particularly when you are in poor health as well as being in poor physical shape.

"Be around for your kids and grandchildren" "health—what's it worth?"

"It is priceless"

You will have to make sometime during the day for your exercise. No, no, don't say that you're too busy. What in the world is your health worth? It doesn't take long to realize that it is priceless. So you might have to split it up, some in the morning and some in the evening, if need to be. Once you remind yourself daily that your health is priceless, you will find the time to get it done. Yes, you will be sure to maintain what you have accomplished, as it is the key to your priceless, healthy life.

We know that prescription drugs have side effects. If we have several things wrong, we could be taking several different drugs, and some take diet pills on top on that. It sure happens, and can you imagine what this does to your poor system? How many people read all the Info about drugs they are taking? Not many, I'm sure. This is not a crusade against prescription drugs as I still take some myself. This is about how to reach and maintain your best health level of your age by following through and doing a few simple things.

It's up to us as individuals to get this done for ourselves and our love ones. Thank you for taking the time to read this, but really, what's more important than your health? I hope my insight on what I have learned over the years, if nothing else, inspires you to take charge of your own wellbeing, as it is up to you.

Yes, no question, you can do it.

## ABOUT ME

I'm not an expert on what you should eat or on the medicines or herbs you should take. The only things that I can tell you are what I have learned and what works for me. I recognize that everyone is different, so some things might not work for you or be healthy for you. Always check with your primary care physician before starting anything new.

'Read on – find out how to maintain 'we are all different check with doctor' 'a real blessing '

For me to have any creditability with you, I had best give you some insight into who I am. Am I someone you should put your trust in? I have owned several businesses over the years and thankfully most have been successful. One small business I have is still going in spite of our slow economy. My main customer has been a real blessing. I have been doing business with them for over 40 years. In that time, I could have lost them a few times, and what a big loss that would have been for both companies. Level heads always prevailed, and we found together that we could overcome any obstacle.

It sure makes a difference when you are working with some very nice people and some friendships that have endured. Over this many years, you sure realize how valuable every customer and business relationship are for your success. Always treat your customers like you want to be treated.

# TAKE CHARGE

So here we are looking for ways to be the best we can be in health, wellness, and fitness, certainly three of the most important words for everyone in this wonderful country of ours. No matter how you feel about the healthcare issue, one thing is certain. We, as individuals, need to take charge of our everyday well-being and get and stay on the right path to be as healthy as we can be. Of course, this is even more important for us senior citizens. No, it's not too late. You can really start at any age. Just be sure and check with your primary care physician first.

"Health wellness fitness" "take charge"
"yes you can do it"

I have been blessed with relatively good health in spite of doing the wrong things for years. Having smoked for approximately 50 years, a couple of packs a day, and also drank too much, I know I'm most fortunate to still be here.

Memories of my childhood are of running and playing all kinds of games we would dream up. Primarily, all were exercise. If you have some of those memories, unlock them so you can put them to use for yourself and your love ones.

Children today, I'm afraid, won't have those memories to fall back on. They spend too much time with TV, computers, video games, and sitting around with no exercise. They don't know the joy we had as we made our own fun, and yes, it was mostly exercise. Yes, we have fallen into a trap for sure. We have a room for TV, many times more than one. We need a room for exercise so we can be sure our children are getting an ample amount of it, as well as ourselves. Really, all you need is corner here or there. we really need to unlock our memories which will help bring us health and wellness. We need to get back to doing some of those kinds of things.

## SHOCK TO SEE

As an 88- year- young man, is it any wonder that I'm so concerned about the wellbeing of many of the citizens of this great country of ours? It seems only yesterday that it was rarity to see an obese person at the store. Now we take it for granted, and there are so many. Our society is now made up of many overweight citizens, many who are diabetic or borderline diabetic. When I was in high school in the 40's, I seldom saw an overweight student or teacher. Obesity is really taken for granted today, and folks, it's scary to see what we are doing to ourselves. I have been close to obesity myself. We are in trouble for sure.

## WEIGHT GAIN & BAD HABITS

When I was in my mid-60, I gained an additional 25 pounds, for a total of approximately 40 pounds more than when I was in my early 30's. By that time, I had high blood pressure, my cholesterol was out of control, and I had aches and pains in my knees and elsewhere.

I had wonderful meals as my wife was a super cook, and then there were those fantastic cakes. I just didn't have the will power to say no.

My doctor suggested that I find some will power as I needed to lose some weight. This made sense, for sure, but what really sealed the idea that I had better be doing something was when I went shopping for some new slacks. Here I was looking at 42 'waist. What a laugh, but for sure, there was no way of getting into a smaller size. At that point, I had no energy and sure didn't feel good. Nor did I look healthy. I knew something had to be done.

"Blood pressure high" "Get with it"
"Smoking, drinking bad combo"

I was still smoking at that time. I had quit probably 5 times. I made it nine months once and then went to a big party with lots of alcohol. I pretty much woke up with a cigarette in my hand the next morning. I was back smoking. Drinking and smoking seem to go hand in hand. It is not good, for sure. Finally, I got down to 2 to 4 cigarettes a day but couldn't seem to get over the hill, so to speak. I was trying everything on the market—patches, gum, and what have you. My wife had already quit, so she was a big help, for sure.

After a few more talks with that guy in the mirror, one day I just said this is it and quit for good. I still used the patches for a few days. What a wonderful thing. It was unbelievable how food tasted, and I could actually breathe some air without smoke in it. I can see why people generally gain weight after they stop smoking. You really need to be involved in other things such as exercising. We know how addictive nicotine is and doing things that have to do with your overall health is a good thing when you're trying to quit. "Check with the guy in mirror"

Several months prior to quitting smoking, I had joined an exercise program that I attended three times a week. It started at six in the morning. It was great and consisted of stretching exercises, which I still use today. Then we would walk and/or jog around the gym. This was a great program and really opened my eyes about how exercise, along with cutting down your food intake, could greatly improve your health. Another big plus was the effect this had on my attitude and outlooks on life. It was simply great to be alive. This program suggested to me by my doctor was really the turning point for me in all aspects of health and wellness. It involved exercise, weight control and your personal well-being.

It was wonderful to see transformation of most of the people who attended on a regular basis. Most had experienced heart attacks or had gone through surgery. A nurse was always in attendance to monitor everyone. It was a real eye-opener for me, getting to know some of the other people and hear what it was like for them and how they felt about the program. One thing was for sure, everyone who attended on a regular basis was very thankful for this program and how it assisted everyone in their recovery. For me, being close to them three days a week really encouraged me to make this work. I feel for sure this program was the turning point for me in my effort to quit smoking. "Opened my eyes" "hope for everyone" "encouraged a turning point"

The name of the program was CAPRI, which is short for Cardio Pulmonary Rehabilitation Institute. What a great program which, a year after I completed the course, lost its funding. This program or maybe something similar might be available in other parts of the country. So, for now, with the shortage of funds for such things, you will need to take things in your own hands and either start your own home exercise program or join a group program, but do it now, not next week or month. You can do it. Get started today. "Time for us to get started" "up to you"

While writing about things that have helped me, I realized that none of this would help anyone unless I talked about the products I have used. It's time we did something about our health and wellness. Do it now. You will be so glad that you did, and you will be on your way to be the best that you can be." You will be glad you did"

## GETTING STARTED

With this background, I wanted to pass on a few thoughts and ideas that have worked for me over the years. There are all kinds of ideas on how to proceed but finding the right things for you is what you should be looking for. The change we are talking about is not only our exercise program but also in our eating habits. One thing that really helps is to have minds—eyes-view of yourself looking and feeling better than you're out of shape body and mind. This gives you something to strive for and to work towards, goal if you will. "Do some stretching" "our minds eye"

For starters, the best idea is just walking after doing some stretching exercises. This will get your whole body into it. Guess what? Walking is free—one of the few things that is. Just thirty minutes each day, for starters, three times a week will make a big difference. Be sure you have the proper footwear, which is even more important if you are overweight. If you look after yourself, it will influence someone else to do the same. It really works this way and helps keep everyone motivated.

Besides, you might end up with a workout partner,

Most people in the know will tell you that walking is the best place to start, and from my own experience, I certainly agree. It would be a waste of time if you went out and injured yourself right away. Remember that your heart, lungs, arms, feet, legs, knees, and all your joints come into play just by walking. It seems like a simple idea, but believe me, it is the best place to start. And yes, it definitely will work for you.

It it's raining out, be sure and grab your umbrella with your walking shoes, or go to the nearby mall, which I have done many times. Or just use your umbrella. Or just stay home and use your at-home exercise equipment, which we will cover in the next chapter. The important thing is continuity. This is of vital importance to your success, so get going. Get started today. You will be so happy that you did. When you start feeling better, you will look back and wonder, "What was I doing to myself the way I was living?" You need to keep that positive picture in mind. If you do, you will be on your way to a better life for you and your loved ones.

"Walking for starters- it works for YOU" "proper shoes" "best way to start" "key is continuity"

Be sure and check with your primary care physician before starting anything new. Remember, you can do it.

## AT-HOME WORKOUTS

Now we will look at some good things that you can do indoors, which are great during any season but particularly great during the winter months. Here's some exercise equipment that is low maintenance, won't break the bank, and will do wonders for you.

Trampolines. Wow! Whenever I thought about a trampoline, I visualized a large one in the back yard that only young people could get onto because of the height. Well, what a find this was for me-a trampoline that is only 42 inches in diameter. It comes with a crossbar to hold onto for safety and is maybe 10 inches in height resting on its own legs. I have been using one for more than sixteen years now. I have it just outside my office door at home, actually in the family room as it doesn't require much room.

So those old excuses just won't work anymore, and we have all used them. "It is raining, it's too hot. It's too cold. It's too late," to name just few. There's just no excuse for not using this for two minutes at a time, three times a day and worked up from there. This gives you a great work out if you swing your arms as if walking or jogging as you bounce. Also they are low impact and are easy on your joints and muscles. NASA says that it is effective for helping astronauts deal with body deterioration from periods of weightlessness in space. It is even better than running, they say. Using the small trampoline/rebounder helps your legs, buttocks, and abs. Many people think that a trampoline could be the best piece of exercise equipment yet devised. Rebounding is a terrific exercise and generally puts you in a state of mental and physical wellness. It will also rejuvenate your body when it's tired. You can find more detail about the rebounder in the section with that title.

"Great exercise equipment "

"What works for me now are three session a day of 8-10 minutes each, at least three times a week" "More effective than running" Another wonderful home exercise machine is the stationary bike. I have one and use it at least three times a week. The bike's values are known worldwide, and what a great job it does in building your leg muscles and your endurance.

"Stationary bike-great leg muscles"

You need to keep a journal of the exercises that you can do each day. We will cover this in detail later on, as it is more important that to make sure this becomes second nature.

I feel better now than I have for 20-some years. I'm not saying this is to brag but only to point out some things we do for ourselves that will help us maintain our good health. These workouts will take care of your waistline. I've been able to maintain what I was striving for, what I'm really pleased with is my blood pressure. It is better than the average I was looking for, and best of all. I've been able to maintain it, these are fun things the whole family can do, even from your own home.

My first week with the trampoline/rebounder, I twisted my ankle as I was just using my everyday shoes. My grandkids might be on there with no shoes, but for us senior citizens, I believe we should have some exercise shoes.

"Feel better-do these for your health and wellness" be sure and check with your primary care physician before starting anything new.

"Be sure and be involved in your children's exercise"

Yes, for sure, you can do it.

## OTHER EXERCISES

It could be tennis, bowling, ice/roller skating, skiing, swimming, soccer, golf, dancing or any number of things. Just make sure that it's something you enjoy doing.

For me its golf a wonderful game that we can play throughout most all of our lives. We hear and read so much about how to improve our swing, but I think the best asset of playing is the mental wellbeing it brings to everyone. From the phone call to or from a friend setting up a date for the next game, the benefits that each person realizes are tremendous. Our psyche receives a big boost which improves our mental health and really helps our physical health as well.

I've also found that my score is way down the list of the real assets of the game. Good thing, too. Just being outside in the fresh air, sunshine, with all the wonderful exercises of practice swings, walking, bending, and kneeling is enough. This is a great game that will do a world of good for everyone. The clubs, shoes, and the golf balls we have today are fantastic, so we are well outfitted. Most of these and maybe other wonderful assets will be true no matter what game or exercise you participate in. The key is to keep yourself in shape so you can continue to enjoy a healthy lifestyle. Yes, you can do it.

"Many wonderful things you do" "get involved "
"great to be outside"

"keep yourself in shape"

Another fun thing I love to do is dance. Now before you dismiss it, please consider this: dancing is one of the great pleasures of life. You and that special someone will have great fun dancing. I try to go twice a week. Listen, you don't need to be ballroom perfect. Even the beginners and those who have not danced in many years have a great time. Everyone has their own style, anyway. I urge you to find a place where you can dance or take dance class, which many people do. They can always tell you where you find places to dance. Believe me; dancing has helped to save many marriages. For sure, dancing is a great exercise, and yes, you can even do this at home. Give it a try. You will love it "dancing - one of the great pleasures"

A combination of healthy mind and body will produce the results you are looking for. Yes, you can make this happen to yourself and your loved ones, so get up and get headed in the right direction. Remember the talk you had with the guy in the mirror.

"Mind and body"

Be sure and check with your primary care physician before starting anything new.

## MENTAL WELLBEING

If you are married or just have the special someone in your life, you will find that these exercises and other ideas will be of value for you. Love and all the wonderful things that go along with it are very important for our mental wellbeing, being in shape, both mind and body, has many rewards for all of us.

"So very important our mental well-being"

If circumstances find you without a special someone in your life, please take heart. There is someone for you.

This is really a key ingredient for our mental health and wellness, our outlook, and mental wellbeing, in the 50's and 60's, your best chance for meeting someone was to go to a bar that had dancing, and there was lots of them at the time. Today, you are hard pressed to find dancing during the week unless you are fortunate enough to belong to a fraternal Organization. Even then, it's more likely to be on the weekend.

"Your special someone"

How fortunate we are today. With just flick of your mouse, you can find someone to just chat with or meet for coffee, tea, or whatever, and chances that you never would have met them otherwise. What a difference the computer has made, as you can even narrow things down to a religious preference. There are really some wonderful people out there. So, this is your chance to help full fill your life. Please, do yourself a favor. Get busy and check out the dating sites that you can find out on the internet. Do it now as this will improve your overall health and wellness.

For sure, having that special someone in your life will help you make the changes and give you the incentive to follow through.

"For your overall mental health, wellness and happiness"

## EXERCISE- MEDICINE- HERBS

In order to keep track of what exercises you are doing and what medicines and herbs you are taking on a daily basis, you need to keep a log. I have been doing this for years now, and it works great. I use a scratch pad for this and put both on the same pad, but you can use whatever method works for you, just do it every day. For exercise, I use the first letter or two of each one and then the amount of time spent on that particular exercise. It sure works for me, and there is a sample of how it looks. You can make as many columns as needed for the medicines and herbs. The codes for your exercises could be as follows, which is how I do it.

"Easy to keep your daily log"

**Exercise Codes:**
- ✓ Bike- B
- ✓ Warm-up- WU
- ✓ Golf-G
- ✓ Walking-W
- ✓ Trampoline/rebound- T
- ✓ Yard work –YW
- ✓ Dancing-D
- ✓ Housework-HW

You also need to make up a code for the medicines and herbs you take. I do this as follows:

### Medicines and herbs- Codes

- ✓ Blood pressures Pill-BP
- ✓ Water pill-WP
- ✓ All-day energy greens- ADEG
- ✓ Vitamins-VH
- ✓ Chlorella-SU

This is what I do. You can set up your own program. Just be sure to do it daily. I keep track of medicine, herbs, and exercises daily. It is easy. Just be sure to do it everyday.

| EXERCISES | | vit | bp | wp | adeg |
|---|---|---|---|---|---|
| Wu - 10 | 11/2 | x | x | x | x |
| W – 25 | | | | | |
| T – 8 / 43 | | | | | |
| Wu - 5 | 11/3 | | | | |
| B - 20 | | x | x | x | |
| t- 10 / 35 | | | | | |
| wu – 8 | 11/4 | | | | |
| yw - 40/48 | | x | x | x | x |
| wu - 10 | 11/5 | | | | |
| w - 28 | | | | | |
| t – 8/46 | | x | x | x | x |

In reality, you post this info in longhand, which is what I do. It was typed so everyone could read it easily.

You probably noticed that under exercise I include yard work. The reason I do this because working in the yard is great exercise which I happen to enjoy. But even if you don't like it much, just consider it as good workout. It makes it easier to do. The same theory can be applied to anything that you do around the house, from painting to vacuuming. It is all great exercise, for sure. Be sure and make exercise a part of your daily routine. We have so much to gain but changing our eating habits, and combined with regular exercise, it will bring out a more cheerful and positive attitude and a much higher energy level.

"Yard work- anything around the house- great exercise"

Maybe the only exercise we will have in common is walking, but the key is to do something to stay on the right track for a healthy and bright life. Don't forget, you can do it.

"Be sure and write it down"

## A FEW REMINDERS

Why is it so important to write our food consumptions and exercise down on a log each day? If you don't do this, you will soon skip a session or two because you are two busy or you don't feel like it that day. If you don't write it down, you will soon be skipping it entirely. Or you will be telling yourself, "I did this the other day, so I'm okay. I've been there and done that." Soon you are not doing it at all.

Here's an interesting statistic: of people that join a health club, after a couple of months, 70% of then have quit. I have nothing against

health clubs, but I have been part of that statistic. We start with good intentions but soon quit, and we're done. Don't do that, please. You must write these down daily. As we get older, exercise gets harder to do and is hard work it if we let it be.

"We start with good intentions"

"Statistics after couple of months 70% quit" "write it down"

Keep that good frame of mind and get it done for your own well-being. Your family will be glad you did, and so will you. Look in the mirror and have a good heart-to-heart talk with that person. Yes, you can do it.

"Frame of mind meant so much"

What we eat really has everything to do with our wellbeing. As I pointed out, I'm certainly no expert on what we should eat or on medicines and herbs we should take. The only thing I can tell you is what works for me, and of course, you should check with your family doctor before you try something new.

"Apples and oranges are great- make them a habit"

I start every day with an apple. I have been doing this for at least 25 years. An apple does so many good things for you, one of which is keeping your digestive system working properly. Probably four times a week, I will also have an orange with it. "Pineapple, cherries, grapes, bananas great for snacks"

➢ **Breakfast:**

At least four times a week, I have a bowl of cooked oatmeal with a spoonful of raisins and maybe one teaspoon of honey. Instead of milk, I use apple juice most of the time. I also add a spoonful of cinnamon. This is a great breakfast. It stays with you and is less than 500 calories. Other days, I will have either scrambled eggs with left over vegetables and one piece of toast or cold cereal, oats, or Great Grains with a sliced banana.

"Oatmeal, great with apple juice"

> **Lunch:**

I have my main meal at noontime as it just seems to work better for me. Then I have a light meal in the evening when I am generally winding down and more apt to be watching TV or reading.

"Noon — main meal"

Most of the time, this main course is fish, other seafood, or chicken. Also, tossed green garden salads are a big part of this meal. I only have beef two or three times a month. Also, I have a glass of V8 juice with my noon meal.

> **Evening:**

At night, I usually will have a bowl of soup or chili with a sandwich of ham and/or turkey. Several times a week, I will have a fruit meal with fresh pineapple, strawberries, grapes, cherries, and half a banana. Then, on another night, I might have an apple, an orange, and some grapes or cherries. Also, I usually have some watermelon around for snack. These fruit meals really fill you up and keep the calories

down. Usually have some veggies cooked up and can also use them in a veggie omelette.

"Try the fruit and veggie meal - always good"

Most important - write everything down on your log.

➢ **Snacks/Desserts:**

You really have to be careful here. Read those labels. We should all be aware of the salt and sugar in most of these snacks. These will cause you a great deal of harm, particularly if you eat them daily. These are the most important for you to write down on your log. The best thing, I have found, is to eat some fruit.

"Loaded - read the labels"

I use a curve of between 1600 and 1850 calories per day. Sometimes, I will be down around 1499 when I eat a lot of fruit and veggies, but I will be well satisfied. Some people will say this won't work, but as I have said, it works for me. So be sure and check with your doctor before starting anything new. This is even more important if you are really out of shape.

"Great stuff for our well-being" Other things I do:

Another thing I do daily is have a cup of herbal or green tea with one plus teaspoons of apple cider vinegar added. This has terrific properties as it has pectin, beta, carotene, potassium, essential amino acids, and healthy enzymes, which some people claim extends our youthfulness. I have been doing this for approximately the last

eight years and drinking tea every day for approximately fifteen years.

"Green tea really great"

I have, in the past, added a spoonful of honey to my tea/vinegar and still do if my digestive system is out of sorts. I do use honey with my oatmeal as honey is wonderful and is about the most perfect food with great healing qualities.

"About the most perfect food"

I started keeping track of what I was eating approximately six years ago. I did this so I could really see what I was consuming daily and what it really looked like over a week's time. It's really simple, and it is a big help for me. You don't seem to forget that piece of cake you had. Put everything down, and then you can spot the changes you need to make in order to get back eating healthy. I just use a scratch pad for this as follows:

"Keep track log it daily - it's a big help"

DATE 12/23/10 - Meals for this date - showing calories consumed

- ➢ Breakfast
- ○ Oatmeal - 150
- ○ Raisins – 65
- ○ Honey – 120
- ○ Apple juice - 60
- ○ Apple - 90 Total: 485

- ➢ Lunch
- ○ Lemon pepper fish - 300 w/ rice and vegs
- ○ V8 juice - 50 Total: 350

- ➢ Dinner
  - Chili – 160
  - Bread – 260
  - Ham & mayo - 90  2cookies - 160  Total: 648

**Total for the day: 1,480**

I do this in long hand on a scratch pad. It is typed here so everyone can read it easily.

## HERBS & SUPPLEMENTS

There are so many wonderful products on the market today. One of the best and one I have been using for years is the product Chlorella. This is a food product first produced in Japan. It is a wholly natural food. It comes in small tablet form. Chlorella is freshwater, single-cell green algae, and it is a nutrient-dense super food. It contains 60% protein, 18 amino acids (including all of the essential amino acids), and various vitamins and minerals. Its deep green comes from extremely high chlorophyll content. I started off with 5 tablets a day after a meal and now take 15 per day, which is what they recommend. This sounds like a lot, but it is only a small tablespoon full. I never miss taking them.

"Great product full of wonderful things our body needs"

Most health food stores carry chlorella products, or you can find informational online about this very fine product and find out who to contact. Follow up and contact them. You will be glad you did.

My wellbeing is certainly due in part to this great product. Here is a wonderful product that I use called energy greens. This super product contains 38 different ingredients including herbs, herbal extracts, grass juice, vitamins, antioxidants, and bioflavonoids. Approximately one tablespoon exceeds the equivalent of 5 national standard servings of vegetables and fruit. Just mix one tablespoon with your favorite juice, and you have a tasty drink that will do wonders for you. I use this at least three times a week. This product also has chlorella in it. My wellbeing is certainly due, in part, to this wonderful product.

"All day energy"

"Equal to 5 servings of fruit and veggies"

Many health food stores carry this product, or you can go online and find energy drinks. Just be sure it has the ingredients that I mentioned. Be sure and follow up as this will help your energy level for sure.

My wellbeing is certainly due, in part, to this wonderful product.

*RJ Smith*

## COST-HERBAL SUPPLEMENTS & EXERCISE EQUIPMENT

I believe it is important to look at what the daily cost to the consumer are, as there are many misconceptions. You hear, "Oh heavens, I can't afford the high cost of herbal supplements or exercise equipment." This has always been a great excuse for not doing anything and continuing on with a life destroying program. So, let's take a look.

These figures are recent as I just made these purchases:

Energy greens - one serving per day: $0.81 per day Chlorella - 15 tablets per day: $1.00 dollar per day

Daily vitamins: $1.00 dollar per day

Some people who say they can't afford these expensive supplements will spend twice this or more per day on pop, candy, and other things they really should stay away from. Look in the mirror and ask yourself, "What is my health worth?"

Let's look at the trampoline. For this example, let's say that it cost $200. The small, in home ones will cost less than this. We will say it has a life of 4 years, but they will last longer than this.

3 times per week x 52 weeks = 156 times per year.

156 times per year x 4 years = 624 times

This works out to $0.32 every time you use it if you used it every day for four years, the cost would be less than $0.14 per day.

This is one of the great bargains for people who are looking to find a better way to improve their health and wellness and their life.

Go back to the mirror and be honest with yourself. "How much money do I spend each day on things that are helping me be a healthy vibrant person, things that I and my loved ones will be very

proud of? I'm ready to make the commitment to make this work for me."

All aspects of your life can and will improve when you pursue a healthy lifestyle. Yes, put some zest in your life. You will glad that you did.

## **MEDICINES-HERBAL ALTERNATIVES**

There are several doctors that write monthly newsletters on health, healing, and alternatives that are available to the public. These newsletters will keep you up to date and ahead of new ideas and products. They are aimed towards prevention and natural therapies. Also, these doctors keep abreast of important findings from around the world. Solutions for some 20 common health problems have been found and reported through these newsletters.

Some of these doctors also produce daily dietary supplements that are loaded with natural vitamins, minerals, and antioxidants. I have used some of them, particularly the daily vitamin products, and find them to be outstanding as they give you that daily advantage. You can find these products at your local health food store, or you can find them online where you can buy them direct and also learn about all of the other products that they offer.

With the healthcare issue still a mess, it is more important than ever that we take the necessary steps to reach and maintain our best health and wellness. We are responsible for our own health. We must make sure that we do the very best for ourselves and our loved ones.

## PUBLICATIONS

Calories:

I have read and refer frequently to some publication. There is one that had pictures of food comparisons with total calories listed for each group. It's great to see these comparisons and it really makes you stop and think about what you are consuming. One particular book was #1 for a time, and it is a must read and has helped me a lot.

Sugar:

All kinds of sugar are a big problem in our daily diet. It seems like everything we eat has some sugar in it, other than the natural ones.

This really can get out of control for any of us but is much easier to spot now that the ingredient list is on everything. There are all kinds of sugar products so it's necessary to keep up to speed on this. There are several books that were #1 best sellers, particularly on what to do with the fat around your middle. Look after yourself and stay abreast of the latest information.

## WARM-UPS

What I do:

1. Touch your fist together in front of your chest, count 1 - 2 -3 as you pump your arms out to each side.
2. Standing up, bend forward at the waist and do the swimming stroke with your arms. Turn your head just as you would if you are swimming. I do 30 of these.
3. Standing up, do the swimming back stroke with your arms. I do 30 of these.
4. Knee bends or squats: place your hands on your hips, and then bend your knees as if sitting. I do 15 of these.
5. Touch your toes. I do 15 of these.
6. Standing, extend your arms to each side and then twist (turn) at the waist. I do 15 of these.
7. Lay on the floor. Raise your legs, ankles together. I do 15 of these.
8. Lay on the floor. Raise your legs. Spread your legs, and then touch your ankles together. I do 15 of these.
9. Lay on the floor. bring your right knee up towards your chest. Hold your knee just below the kneecap with both hands and

pull towards your chest, counting 1-2-3-pull. Release slightly, then do the same with the left leg. I do 15 with each leg.
10. Hand weights, 10lbs each: I do some over the head as well as holding them straight to the side and lifting. Also, you can do this straight out in front of you.

Remember, this is what I do, which might not be the right thing for you. There are all kinds of exercises, and you need to find what is best for you. Be sure and check with your primary care physician before doing any of these or others.

## TRAMPOLINES/REBOUNDERS

Here are some powerful reasons to have and use a trampoline/rebounder, and there are many:

- Increased circulation
- Strengthening of pelvic floor muscles which help control stress
- Stimulating of metabolism
- Lowering elevated cholesterol and triglyceride levels
- Strengthening around your joints without putting pressure on them
- Burning approximately 300 calories per hour
- You can watch movie while using it
- Enhanced digestion
- Dramatically lowered incidence of stroke and heart disease
- Reduced blood pressure
- Help in maintaining peak brain function

- Aids in muscle tone and performance "great way for getting your kids involved- they will love it" "great for all ages"

Caution: if you are going to purchase one, be sure that it has the stabilizing bar, as sometime during my exercise I need the bar to

maintain my balance. The company I bought mine from is no longer in business, but there are plenty of companies that sell them. Some now come with several stabilizing bars on them plus some netting, probably to protect small children from falling off. "Used by astronauts - found to be a great fitness tool"

NASA, through their studies, has shown that rebounding Is actually 68% more effective as a fitness conditioner compared to running and other forms of aerobic exercise?

There are so many ways that a trampoline is a wonderful tool for at-home exercise:

You can have one in your home, and it only has a 42" diameter, a very small space. Many people just don't have the time to drive to an exercise facility. Even if you do have the time, consider this. Let's say you have a one-hour window. If you have to drive, and even if it's close by, say fifteen minutes each way, which includes getting in and out of your garage and walking in and out of the facility, this leaves you 30 minutes for a workout. Compare that to having a trampoline/rebounder at home. You could do 3 sessions of 8-10 minutes each and have 10-12 minutes rest between each session, plus time to warm-up. An hour is hard to find, particularly if you have children. This makes for a great home workout, rain or shine.

Men, the trampoline/rebounder has some fantastic benefits for you. As you know, a man's libido starts to decline before he reaches 40. One of the things that happens as we age are not getting enough exercise, so consequently, our blood circulation slows down. Using a rebounder on a regular basis will not only help keep your weight under control, it will do wonders for your circulation.

This is really one of a kind and does so many great things for your body and also your mind, because you will feel and look healthy, so be sure and give this a try. It won't break the bank either. Happy jumping.

## CALORIES

You can find lots of information about calories. Some good articles on calories can be found at www.idealweightcharts.com/caloriecounterchart.html.

Also, the food guide pyramid gives you all kinds of information on food groups and dietary guidelines. Be sure and pay attention to what you are consuming. You want to use these guides as an outline for what to eat each day. The pyramid calls for eating a variety of foods to get the nutrients you need; this will assure you that you are eating the right number of calories to maintain your weight. The focus should be on fat as most diets are too high in fat, especially saturated fat. Some nutrition materials, the food guide pyramid graphic, and the Dietary Guidelines for Americans may be accessed thru the CNPP home page at http:/www.usda.gov/fcs/cnpp.htm.

## **BRAIN-BODY CONNECTION**

Once in a while in life, we learn about something new that we can't help talking about and telling friends and loved ones about, which is how I feel about the upper cervical chiropractic health care procedure.

I first heard about the brain-body connection when I heard the radio program of a doctor in the Seattle area. I was really impressed by what I heard and was soon making it a habit to tune in whenever possible on Sunday at noontime.

One of the first things the doctor explained is what upper cervical health care is about, and he made it clear that he does not heal, as it is the body itself that does the healing. What the doctor is able to do is put the head and body into proper alignment so they can work together and allow the healing process to begin. According to the doctor the head weighs 10 to 14 pounds which is basically the size of a bowling ball, all the nerves from the brain come down at the back of the neck into the spinal column. When your head is not in balance with your body, caused when the atlas (first bone in the neck) is set at a slight tilt, some nerves will become pinched. What we have then are aches and pains, which can really have an adverse effect on our everyday life, which will grow worse until proper communication is restored. The doctor's thorough exam includes some x-rays of the neck and spine area, which he analyzes so he can determine if he can help you with that.

My wonderful lady had been having back and knee problems and was seeing a chiropractor a couple of times a month. Sometimes she would be fine for a week, and other times it might be the next day when she would be in pain again. Approximately 3 years ago, she developed what we called musical ear. I'm not sure who came up with the name. She would hear different songs, every verse, which lately had been virtually 24/7. Some of the music she hadn't heard in years, and the volume would become increasingly louder each day. She had many nights with little sleep and even questioned her sanity, especially after some specialists told her she probably would just have to live with it.

Every time I would hear this radio program, I became convinced this method would help her if anything could. After she heard the program a few times, with all the testimonials, she was convinced she should try it and made an appointment. Of course, I had to go along.

At the first appointment, the doctor explained what the upper cervical health care method is about and how it works so your body can start the healing process. Next he found out from her what her history had been as far as any injuries she might have sustained, what problems she had, and all symptoms including when they started and what she had done to relieve any pain, etc. He then took some pictures of her neck and back so he could analyze them. After doing so, he said he felt he could help her and pointed out the areas that were out of alignment. He had no idea if this would help her musical ear, but her body would be in proper alignment, which would help her other problems. On the third appointment, he went over everything she had told him, in detail— he didn't miss a thing. He then made this first adjustment. She could hardly tell he had done anything, as it wasn't painful at all; he knew just how much pressure to apply.

She says it is a miracle. Her knee pain is gone, her back is 90 percent better than it has been, and the musical ear is virtually gone. She has heard it for only a few minutes, and then it was very soft. She is now able to sleep, as musical ear hasn't bothered her at night.

It is truly amazing. This treatment has worked for many different problems, from vertigo, panic attacks, and it now looks like musical ear can be added to the list. It has now been over two months, and she is doing great.

I took a bad fall when I was sixteen. I fell approximately six feet and landed on my tailbone before going another five feet to the ground. I developed cysts on my tailbone and, over the next eighteen months, had several hospital stays before these would heal up. For years I have had back, hip, and knee problems, probably due to this fall. I have seen many doctors and chiropractors over the years, and at best, the relief has been only temporary. I have been told many times I have one leg shorter than the other but have been given no solutions to correct it. Using the upper cervical process, this is one of the main clues that your body is out of balance. So I had all the tests done, which showed that my body was out of alignment, and this was one time I'm really looking forward to my next doctor's appointment. By the afternoon of my first appointment, the pain in my right knee had virtually disappeared and my hips were much better by the next day. It is now going in two months, and my follow ups have all been good. We have been able to maintain my alignment correction. The healing process continues, and I have continued my preventative maintenance program and everything is going well.

This is certainly the best-kept health care secret that I have ever seen and a great plus for everyone with no surgery and no prescription drugs. Look for chiropractors who used the upper cervical health care method, as this procedure can really help you toward a full life of health and wellness.

## IN CONCLUSION

Each of us has to take charge of our own well-being by eating and exercising as we should. Your family will be so thankful, or maybe your whole family needs to make some changes. If so, then the sooner you make the changes, the better, certainly. Just think, this could mean a completely different and wonderful life, compared to what would have been had you continued on a health-destroying lifestyle. Naturally, our children will be eating and exercising as we do, and if we are doing the wrong things, then sometime down the road this will show up as more prescription drugs to keep us going or maybe as a precursor to obesity or diabetes. We would not do this to ourselves or our loved ones deliberately, so we need to think about it now and make the necessary changer. We all know how time flies, and it's so easy to put off. This has to be priority number one, not number 10, which is more than likely going to get put off to some other time.

Heart disease is still the number one killer, brought on in many cases by our poor eating habits and lack of exercise. We need to do this with a team effort and support the ones who are doing the right things.

With the great abundance of food, exercise equipment, and facilities in our country, there really is no excuse. Hopefully, I have awakened your concerns about your health and wellness so that you will start doing something about it.

We must make some changes in what we eat by cutting as much sugar, salt, and refined carbohydrates as we can. Exercise as many muscles as you can by varying your exercises some. Think about it. Put it in motion. Write it down daily in your log.

Yes, you can do it, and you will look forward to being the best you can be. It's time to get started. You really have so much to look forward to, through healthy eating and exercise. Your main goal should be to be physically fit for your age, which includes a healthy heart, blood pressure, and cholesterol and a weight in a good range. This is not an impossible goal. You can do it. I can't stress enough how very important exercise is for the success of this program. So get up and get started on being the best you can be, and don't forget to log what you have done each day. There are many herbal supplements to help you control your weight and improve your wellbeing. Be sure and contact these companies and ask for further information on their products to see if they have something you can use. My good health and wellness are due in part to the wonderful herbal supplements that I use. Excess weight or obesity is the biggest contributor to nearly every health problem. It is now known that it can worsen colon cancer, breast cancer, and prostate cancer, and it also has an effect on arthritis, sleep problems, and even ED and infertility. Diabetes is epidemic in our country. Nearly 26 million have it, and approximately 7 million are undiagnosed and aren't being treated. Then there are nearly 80 million people who are pre-diabetic and are at the highest risk of developing the disease. It is imperative that we form new eating habits along with an exercise program. As I have mentioned, the best way to start is to just walk and team up with someone. As this helps keep everyone motivated. It really works that way. Also, be sure and keep your daily log of food that you consume and exercises that you do. It has been proven that people who do this lose twice as much weight as those who don't. If you splurge or miss a day, just get yourself back on track. Yes, you can do it and be the best that you can be.

## Motivation:

When I see people smoking, I wonder what they are thinking. Don't they realize that they are destroying their health and maybe headed toward lung cancer, heart problems, or some other life- threatening problem? Well, you know, it's the same thing if you are overweight or obese. You are destroying your health, maybe even faster than the smoker. Just look where you are heading- maybe right into diabetes, heart problems, or some other life- threatening problem.

So yes, it's time to look in the mirror and have a heart to - heart with that person. Ask yourself, "What is my health and wellness worth?" Some people find motivation in the fear of some of their doctor's forecasts coming through if they don't change their ways. Others are drawn to the outdoors for their love of an activity they did as young person. Yes, we need to open those memory banks and return to doing some physical activity. Regular physical activity is the most important thing we can do for ourselves, no matter what our age. Find your motivation. Envision how you'll achieve your goals. Be strong. Yes, you can do it, and you can be headed for the best you can be. There are many good articles and books so be sure and get the help you need.

## Will power:

Change your daily habits to something that is new. You'll be doing that very thing when you start your new eating and exercise program. So now that you have a new routine, maybe add an early evening walk. You then can allow yourself to do your favorite thing. There are many articles on will power, so be sure and read up on how to make this work for you. You can make this work along with your new program of health, wellness and fitness. Yes, it is so very important, and you can do it.

## Longevity:

In a recent study of 17 developed countries, it was shown that US men ranked last and US women next to last. It has been known for some time that the US fares poorly in comparison with other rich countries. Most studies have focused on older age when the most people die.

This report showed that deaths before age 50 accounted for two thirds of the difference in life expectancy between US males and their counterparts in other developed countries and approximately one third of the differences for females. Even discounting that deaths from car accidents, gun violence, and drug overdoses, the US has long lagged in life expectancy compared with other economically developed countries. Unfortunately, we have very damaging, unhealthy behaviors. No matter how you feel about our health care situation, it is way past time for us, as individuals, to take responsibility for our own health and wellness. It behooves us to think about our health on a daily basis as our time on this earth is so fleeting. A good many of us have visited someone in a nursing home, and while the facilities continue to improve, that is the last place we wish to end up. In our senior years, we certainly want to be the best we can be. It is up to us.

What goes on between your ears has a lot to do with your longevity as you can stimulate and control it.

Good health, which extends your life, begins with a body that is maintained by good eating with exercises that lead to health and wellness. A healthy body needs a diet with an assortment of nutrients and other elements. When shopping, be sure and do more shopping in the live food section for those fresh fruits and vegetables. This is true no matter what diet you might be on. Also, remember that the natural sugars from the fruit tend to go straight to your blood streamed, where they help regulate your blood or are sent out of your system. We sure know what refined sugars will do, especially in the amounts we tend to consume. Illnesses over 50 are degenerative diseases such as cancer, heart attacks, and strokes which are affected by whatever we eat and how we live. Control some of your future by what you eat and how much exercise you get. You have just one body, so be sure and take care of it.

Using preventive maintenance, you soon will radiate good health and wellness. Yes, you can do it and be the best that you can be. My program is for everyone, as it's never too late to start taking care of yourself. While my program is for everyone, my main intent is to help prevent diabetes and obesity, so we therefore need to start with our children as early as possible, teaching them to practice good nutrition and exercise. With today's lifestyle of more TV and computer time, along with less exercise in the schools, it is imperative that we teach ourselves and our children that good nutrition and exercise are the most important things we can do for ourselves.

If not, we could face a lifetime of health problems, and becoming senior citizen would be a thing of the past. Yes, you can do it and be the best that you can be. I use the following foods/condiments, many of them several times a day. These are favorites of mine and have certainly contributed to my good health and wellness. They will have wonderful properties, and I believe we should all take a closer look at them.

Remember, these are foods I use, and while they have been wonderful for me, they might have an adverse effect on you, particularly if you are on certain medications. So check with your family doctor to be sure that you can proceed. In any case, I have found it is best to start slow with small quantity for starters.

## Garlic:

Garlic has been found to be one of the best remedies for blocking cancer of the stomach, pancreas, breast, prostate, lungs, kidneys, and brain. When you chop up, mash, or however you prepare your garlic, keep it away from heat for at least 10 minutes so the garlic will retain its medical benefits. By not waiting those 10 minutes, approximately 90% of the antioxidants could be destroyed. I have found that garlic is great with most foods including using it on sandwiches and putting some in my soup, salads, and hot dishes. It is also wonderful on a bake potato. Try it. Apple cider vinegar:

Apple cider vinegar is an effective bacteria-fighting agent that contains many minerals and elements such as potassium, calcium, magnesium, phosphorus, Sulphur, copper, iron, and silicon that are vital for a healthier body.

Apple cider vinegar is great for the following problems: weight loss, skin problems and infections, constipation, diarrhea, and diabetes, as it helps control high-blood-sugar levels.

I use one to two teaspoons of cider vinegar with my tea several times a day as it helps keep my pH in the correct range and also helps to keep my cholesterol under control.

Some people say that it also will stop your hair from thinning out. After I shampoo, I use it as a rinse on my hair and face, with two teaspoons in a cup of warm water several times a week. Be careful not to get it in your eyes. Men, it is great after shaving as it's an astringent and really makes your face feel great. You will need to experiment to see how much is right for you.

Also, apple cider vinegar is great for washing fruit such as strawberries. Use one-part vinegar to 10 parts cold water for an approximately 15 minutes. This will help take care of the bacteria that might be on our fruits and vegetables.

Vinegar has so many uses. Don't be without it. Buy natural apple cider vinegar with an ideal acidity of 5 percent.

## Cinnamon:

Using cinnamon can lead to dramatic improvements in blood sugar, cholesterol, and triglycerides levels. You can use this so many ways with your meals. I put a couple spoonful on my oatmeal as it blends in very well and makes for a delicious breakfast, and I also use cinnamon on my piece of toast with small amount of honey finished off with some cinnamon. Delicious. Use your imagination as you can use cinnamon so many ways.

There are many claims made for cinnamon, here are some of them:

- ✓ Lowers blood sugar
- ✓ Kills bacteria

- ✓ Improves digestion
- ✓ Reduces inflammation
- ✓ Staves off Alzheimer's diseases

Some researchers claim cinnamon will help control diabetes and others say that not enough studies have been done as of yet. In any case, try it and follow up on continuing studies that are done. Check with your doctor before making changes, particularly if you are on medications.

## Tea:

I usually drink 3-4 cups a day of green tea, topped off with a teaspoon of cider vinegar. I think it's great and does many good things for me, my energy level is great and I feel sure some of this has to do with

tea. Real world evidence is still out on many of these findings. Here are some of the claims about green tea.

- ✓ Great for fighting skin cancer Protects the heart
- ✓ Lowers LDL
- ✓ Lowers blood pressure
- ✓ Protects against diabetes Guards against hepatitis

And there are many more. One question is how much green tea would you need to drink in order to reap its health benefits?

Tea, whether hot or cold, contains powerful antioxidants. It can be green, black, or white. For me, it has been part of my daily routine and is partly responsible for my good health and wellness. Be sure and follow up to keep abreast of all new findings about green tea and tea in general.

Be sure and check with your doctor.

I'm most thankful for the doctor who told me about the CAPRI program. Also, many thanks to my family doctor who encourage me to continue on as I pursued a healthier lifestyle. Losing weight and continuing an exercise program was a good thing for me. I did improve my blood pressure and cholesterol and reduced my weight by doing these things that I have mentioned. From the beginning, I put together some ideas which really worked for me on an ongoing basis. You can do it as you have the power to control and improve your own health by doing the necessary things.

We have a responsibility to take the steps to improve and then maintain our health and wellness. Stay with it. Log it every day, both food and exercise. Be patient and be determined, as it won't happen overnight. Soon, YOU will have something to be proud of for sure. Put some effort into it, and YOU will be rewarded.

One wonderful health care procedure I only recently found is the upper cervical chiropractic health care procedure. This has done wonders for me. You will find, once your body balance has been corrected, this will go a long way toward restoring your health and wellness. I urge everyone to visit with an upper cervical health care doctor, as the test are easy and non-invasive. This is certainly one of the best-kept health care treatments. It is a work in progress, one that takes continued vigilance and is certainly not to be taken for granted. We must take care of ourselves as best we can, not only in minds but also in body.

I'm now nearly 89 years old, and I have reached my goals of losing some weight and improving my blood pressure and my overall health. I have been successful as my averages continue to be:

      **Blood pressure:**      138/74 average
      **Pulse:**      76 average
      6' height, 185 lbs. average, 36" waist

I have found I can maintain this by doing the following things:

- Stretching: approximately 15 minutes per day
- Walking: approximately 1-2 miles per day
- Exercises: rebounder, 3-4 times per week, 8-10 minutes each
- Stationary bike: a couple times per week, 8-10 minutes each

## Meals/Food:

I start each day with a good breakfast which includes plenty of fruit, always an apple, along with maybe an orange, grapes, or other, in-season fruit. I always have my main meal at noon time as this works best for me and probably would for everyone if we would think about it for a minute. You know, generally we are just sitting at night with schoolwork, TV, computer time, or reading which doesn't help our digestive system at all, particularly after a large meal.

I'm careful not to consume too much of the following:

- Salt: check the labels as it seems most things have sodium in them. I try and stay around 2000 mg per day. I use very little from the shaker. Also, check your store as there seem to be new low sodium items every week.
- Sugar: I don't use sugar, not even the artificial type. Use at your own discretion.
- Butter: I use Smart Balance, which is a buttery spread made from vegetable oils.

I continue to use, on a daily basis, garlic, apple cider vinegar, cinnamon and tea.

This is what works for me. As I have stated many times, always check with your doctor before starting any new program.

I has been a learning experience that has been very successful for me, and my hope is that you can find some beneficial ideas that will assist you and give you motivation to be the best you can be, which will have as its reward a healthy life that has longevity with it. Good health is wonderful feeling, and it is something we need to cherish and protect. YES, YOU CAN DO IT.

In this stressful time, it is so very important to stay physically fit and mentally sharp, which will help override the daily problems that might come up.

There are so many ways to lose weight, but more often than not, it is put back on. With his program, once you have reached your goals, it is comforting to know that you will be able to maintain them. My secret to success is simply to continue on with this program and stay aware of what you consume which, along with your exercises, will bring you newfound health and wellness. Look in the mirror. YOU will see a person who has really accomplished something YOU and you loved ones can be very proud of. YOU won't quit your new lifestyle just because you reached your goals. No way. YOU will continue on because feeling and looking healthy is a wonderful thing. Besides, maintaining what YOU have is very easy and enjoyable. You won't just throw it away. So be sure and use your log daily and write it down. By now, it should be second nature and easy to do.

Yes, you have accomplished so much as you have answered the question, "What is my health worth?" Without question, the answer is PRICELESS.

Always keep those positive thoughts, and YOU will be able to look forward to a healthy, full life where you can be the BEST YOU CAN BE.

My best to you, and I will look forward to hearing about your success.

*RJ Smith Head Maintenance Man*

The information and statement made in this publication have not been evaluated by the FDA. The ideas I discussed and recommended are not intended to diagnose, treat, cure or prevent any disease. Individual results may vary. Seek the advice of your health care professional for questions or concerns regarding your health condition and/or needs. The information given here is designed to help you make informed decisions about your body and health.

The suggestions for specific foods, nutritional supplements, and exercises in this program are not intended to replace appropriate or necessary medical care.

Before starting any exercise program, always see your physician first. If you have specific medical symptoms, consult your physician immediately. If any recommendations given in this program contradict your physician's advice, be sure and consult him or her before proceeding. Mention of specific products, companies, organizations, or authorities in this book does not imply that they endorse this book. The author and the publisher disclaim any liability or loss, personal or otherwise, resulting from the procedures in this program.

Internet addresses and phone numbers given in this book were accurate at the time we went to press. Product pictures and trademark names are used throughout this book to describe and inform various property products owned by others. The presentation of such pictures and information is intended to benefit the owner of the product and trademarks and is not intended to infringe upon trademark, copyright, or other rights, or to imply any claim to the mark other than that made by owner. No endorsement of the information contained in this book has been given by the owners of such products and trademarks, and no such endorsement is implied by the inclusion of pictures or trademarks in this book.

www.ingramcontent.com/pod-product-compliance
Lightning Source LLC
Chambersburg PA
CBHW070035040426
42333CB00040B/1688